HERBAL ANTIBIOTICS

FOR BEGINNERS

Your Path to Natural Healing

Disclaimer

A Quick View of the Book

Herbal antibiotics have long been used to treat minor ailments and diseases. Herbs and medicinal plants were the only source of cure in ancient era; that is, before the advancement of medical science. Being said that, it is not only pharmaceutical medical science that has advanced to an unimaginable extent. Herbal medicine has also emerged as a fully fledged field.

As a matter of fact, herbal medicines are normally preferred more to ward off minor illnesses such as cough, cold, external injuries and so on. The increasing awareness about the side effects of pharmaceutical medicines have led people to switch to the less harmful herbal alternative cure, in cases when possible. This book tells you which diseases can be cured by herbal medicines, and it entails quite a number of recipes too.

The "Herbal Antibiotics for Beginners" contains the following:

1. 50 recipes to make a diverse range of herbal antibiotics

2. Every recipe contains a description that tells you the diseases that it can cure, the appropriate dosage and cautions, if any, to be taken.

3. There are recipes to treat cough, colds, infections, wounds, flu, congestion and much more.

4. An entire section is devoted to the recipes of herbal syrups and tonics for cough and cold, influenza and other ailments; and then there is a section for herbal balms and ointments too.

5. You will find an uncountable number of recipes to ease stomach ache and indigestion.

So don't just stop here. Keep on reading to find your path to natural healing!

Contents

Why Do I Need Herbal Alternatives?

An antibiotic may be defined as a medical agent that wards off bodily bacteria and treats the diseases caused by them. However, not all diseases are caused by bacteria. Ailments such as colds, cough, flu, minor infections and other not-so-severe diseases are normally caused by viruses. In such cases, antibiotics are not a healthy cure. Firstly, they may not be that effective; secondly, taking antibiotics too often may cause antibiotic resistance.

Antibiotic Resistance is a phenomenon that is caused as a result of antibiotic overuse. What happens is that when you start taking too many antibiotics, even when the ailment can be cured otherwise, your body gets immune to antibiotics hence rendering them ineffective in times when you really need them.

This book helps you to save your body from being antibiotic resistant. The upcoming section contains herbal recipes to treat a diverse range of diseases. From fever to flu, cough, cold, external wounds, infections, pain, congestions and so on, there is a recipe for almost every minor ailment.

Anti Allergic Nettle Tea

This tea features anti-inflammatory and anti-allergic properties. It is great to treat allergies caused by sneezing, itchy eyes and cold.

Things Needed

2 tsp stinging nettle

1 quart water

1 tsp allspice

Honey, to taste (optional)

Few drops of fresh lemon juice

Procedure

1. Bring the quart of water to boil over a medium-low flame.

2. When the water is fully boiled, turn off the flame.

3. Add nettle to the hot water. Cover and let soak for 20 minutes.

4. Pass the tea through a strainer.

5. Drink all of it throughout the day.

6. Add honey and lemon just before drinking it.

Soothing Anise Tea

This tea is great at treating congestion caused by allergies, cough, cold and flu. It is also good at soothing upset stomachs.

Things Needed

2 tsp crushed anise seeds

Honey, to taste (optional)

1 quart water

Few drops of fresh lemon juice

Procedure

1. Bring the quart of water to boil over a medium-low flame.

2. When the water is fully boiled, turn off the flame.

3. Add the anise seeds to the hot water. Cover and let soak for 20 minutes.

4. Pass the tea through a strainer.

5. Drink all of it throughout the day.

6. Add honey and lemon just before drinking it.

Joint Pain Brew

This is the one of the most effective herbal medicine to treat joint pain.

Things Needed

2 lemons, juiced, reserve the peel

5 quarts water

2 ¼ cups raw sugar

2 lbs nettle tops

1 oz. cream of tartar

1 oz. live yeast

Procedure

1. Bring the water to a boil over a medium-low flame.

2. Add nettle tops to the boiling water. Cook for 15 minutes.

3. Pass through a strainer.

4. Now take a deep skillet or a crock pot and combine the sugar, lemon peel, cream of tartar and lemon juice in it.

5. Add the nettle water to the crock pot.

6. When the water cools down to slightly warm, dissolve the yeast in a little water and then add it to the crock pot.

7. Cover the pot with several folds of cloth and then let it brew for four full days.

8. Strain and discard the residue.

9. You can drink it within 12 days.

Cough and Cold Solution

This solution is very effective in the treatment of cough, cold, bronchitis and asthma.

Things Needed

> 1 tbsp dried basil leaves
>
> 1 tsp ginger powder
>
> Honey, to taste (optional)
>
> 1 quart water
>
> Few drops of fresh lemon juice

Procedure

1. Bring the quart of water to a boil over a medium-low flame.

2. When the water is fully boiled, turn off the flame.

3. Add the basil leaves and ginger powder to the hot water. Cover and let soak for 15 minutes.

4. Pass the liquid through a strainer. Discard the residues.

5. Drink all of it throughout the day.

6. Add honey and lemon just before drinking it.

The Homemade Saline Solution

This makes a simple saline solution that can be used to treat nasal irrigation caused by colds, dryness, allergies and frequent use of nasal sprays.

Things Needed

¼ tsp sea salt

¼ tsp baking soda

8 oz water (about 1 cup)

Procedure

Mix well all the three ingredients and your homemade saline solution is ready to use.

The Herbal Analgesic Compress

The Herbal Analgesic Compress is great at relieving pain that is caused by a sprained joint. It also eases arthritic pain. When used on the chest, it aids in relieving congestion.

Things Needed

4 cups water

2 large bay leaves

1 large piece of wash cloth

Procedure

1. Pour water in a saucepan with a tight fitting lid.

2. Bring the water to boil over a medium flame and then lower the flame to simmer.

3. Add the bay leaf to the simmering water.

4. Cover the pan and let sit for 10 minutes.

5. Discard the bay leaf.

6. Allow the bay leaf water to cool down a little, keep it as hot as you can tolerate on your skin.

7. Now take a clean wash cloth and soak it in this water.

8. Wring out the excess water and press the cloth on the affected area.

9. When the cloth gets cold, re-soak and re-apply.

Herbal Treatment for Congestion

This makes a swallow able paste that is a great medicine to treat cold, cough and lung congestion. It also helps to clear phlegm out of the body

Things Needed

1 tsp of honey

½ tsp of ground black pepper

Procedure

1. Mix well both the ingredients.

2. Swallow the paste with a cup of warm herbal tea or warm water.

Bleeding Control Compress

You can apply this compress to stop bleeding.

Things Needed

1 tsp of yarrow tincture

Half cup of warm water

A piece of soft and clean cloth

Procedure

1. Combine water and yarrow.

2. Soak the cloth in it.

3. Wring out the excess water and press the cloth with a slight pressure on the wounded area.

Cinnamon Gargle

If you have a sore throat or infection in the mouth or gums, gargle at least one time daily with this solution.

Things Needed

½ tsp of ground cardamom

½ tsp of ground cinnamon

1 cup of water

Procedure

1. Bring the water to a boil over a medium-low flame.

2. When the water is fully boiled, turn off the flame.

3. Add the cardamom and cinnamon to the hot water. Cover and let sit for 15 - 20 minutes.

4. Pass the liquid through a strainer.

5. Allow it cool down to warm then use it to gargle.

Indigestion Tea

As the name implies, this tea is great at relieving indigestion. It also aids in the treatment of sore throat and lung congestion.

Things Needed

4 cups of water

1 tsp of ground cardamom seeds

¼ tsp of ground pepper

2 cloves of garlic, ground

½ tsp of ginger powder (substitute: 1 tsp freshly grated ginger)

½ tsp of ground cinnamon

½ tsp of ground coriander seed

Honey, to taste (optional)

Procedure

1. Except for honey, combine all the other ingredients in a saucepan.

2. Cover the pan and simmer for 15 - 20 minutes.

3. Pass the tea through a strainer.

4. Drink it throughout the day.

5. Add honey just before drinking.

Herbal Sanitizer

Using this recipe, you can make your personal homemade hand sanitizer.

Things Needed

1 tsp rubbing alcohol

1 cup of Aloe Vera gel

10 drops tea tree essential oil (substitute: lavender essential oil)

2 tsp vegetable glycerin

Procedure

1. Combine all the ingredients.

2. Keep stored in an airtight bottle.

Herbal Treatment to Leg Syndrome

This makes a relaxing and sweet-tasting remedy to treat restless leg syndrome.

Things Needed

1 tsp of Apple Cider vinegar

1 tsp honey

1 cup water

Procedure

1. Warm the water.

2. Stir in the vinegar and honey.

3. Mix and drink immediately!

Lemonade to Treat Congestion

This drink is great at curing fevers, sore throats and congestion.

Things Needed

½ lemon, juiced

2 tsp honey

1 cup boiling water

Dash of cayenne pepper

Procedure

1. Combine all the ingredients in a mug.

2. Mix well and drink hot.

3. If you are taking it to treat fever, wrap yourself up in a blanket while or immediately after drinking it. This will stimulate the cayenne to cause sweating, and hence break the fever.

Clove Remedy

This recipe makes a clove tea which is great at soothing sore throats and treating cold and flu.

Things Needed

8 cloves of garlic, crushed

1 cup of water

½ tsp of ground black pepper

Honey, to taste

½ tsp of dried ginger

Procedure

1. Bring water to a boil over a medium-low flame.

2. Add the crushed garlic and simmer on low flame for 15 minutes.

3. Stir in the dried ginger and black pepper. Simmer for 2 more minutes.

4. Pass the tea through a strainer.

5. Add honey just before drinking it.

Herbal Treatment for Bloating

This tea is very effective in the treatment of indigestion and bloating. It also helps soothe upset stomach and relieve gas.

Things Needed

2 cups of water

½ tsp of ground coriander

Dash of cayenne pepper

½ tsp of ground cumin

Procedure

1. Bring water to a boil over a medium-low flame.

2. When the water is fully boiled, turn off the flame.

3. Add coriander, cumin and cayenne to the hot water. Cover and let soak for 15 - 20 minutes.

4. Pass the tea through a strainer.

5. Drink warm.

Anti-Gas Remedy

This recipe makes Dill tea which contains anti-gas and sedative properties. It soothes the stomach and is very effective in treating indigestion. The great thing about this tea is that it is safe for children as well. It is extremely effective and widely used to treat common ailments among children including cough, colic, indigestion, gas, insomnia and stomachache.

For kids having colic, a 2 - 4 oz. dosage of the dill weed tea four times a day can get rid of colic. For younger kids, you can give one teaspoon every hour till the excruciating colic pan subsides.

Things Needed

8 oz. water

1 tsp of dill weed (or 1 tsp dill seeds)

Procedure

1. Bring water to a boil over a medium-low flame.

2. When the water is fully boiled, turn off the flame.

3. Add dill weed to the hot water; if you are using dill seeds, rub the seeds and then put them in the boiling water.

4. Cover and let sit for 10 minutes, 15 - 20 minutes if you are using dill seeds.

5. Pass the tea through a strainer.

Treatment for Eye infection

This recipe uses the Eyebright, an herb known for its anti-bacterial and astringent properties. It soothes pink eye and other mild eye irritation and infections. You can use the Eyebright water as an eyewash or as en eye compress.

Things Needed

1 cup of water

1 tsp of dried eyebright herb

Procedure

1. Bring water to boil over a medium-low flame.

2. When the water is fully boiled, turn off the flame.

3. Add the dried eyebright herb to the hot water.

4. Cover and let sit for 10 minutes.

5. Pass it through a strainer

6. Allow it to cool completely.

7. Use it as an eyewash four times a day.

You can also use the Eyebright water as a compress. To do so, perform steps 1 - 5, then allow to become lukewarm. Soak a soft clean cloth in it, wring out the excess water and apply it gently to the affected eye. Leave the compress on eyes for 10 minutes.

Raspberry Leave Tea

The Raspberry Leave Tea works wonders on the female muscles and organs. It is also good for nursing mothers.

Things Needed

2 tsp red raspberry leaves (substitute: 2 red raspberry leaf tea bags)

1 quart of water

1 tsp of ground fennel seeds

Procedure

1. Bring water to boil over a medium-low flame.

2. When the water is fully boiled, turn off the flame.

3. Add the raspberry leaves/raspberry leaf tea bags to the hot water.

4. Cover and let sit for 30 minutes.

5. Pass it through a strainer.

6. Drink all of it throughout the day.

7. You can drink it warm or iced, it is your choice.

Homemade Tranquilizer

This tea is sure to give you a peaceful goodnight's sleep, especially if you have insomnia. Drink this before going to bed.

Things Needed

1 lemon, juiced

2 Tbsp of brandy

¼ cup of water

¼ cup of maple syrup

Procedure

1. Bring water to boil over a medium-low flame.

2. When the water is fully boiled, turn off the flame.

3. Stir in the lemon juice, brandy and maple syrup.

4. Drink warm.

Head Lice Shampoo

This recipe makes a chemical-free homemade and completely herbal anti-lice shampoo.

Things Needed

12 drops of tea tree oil

12 oz. extra virgin olive oil

8 drops of oregano oil

12 drops of rosemary oil

Procedure

1. Combine all the ingredients. Mix well.

2. Apply into hair and scalp.

3. Leave on for 30 minutes then rinse.

4. Repeat this two times a day, till your hair is free of lice.

Ear Ache Remedy

This oil is a great remedy to ease ear ache and infections. You can also use this oil to massage around the ears and neck to relax the lymph nodes and reduce the probability of bacterial infections.

Things Needed

Half cup of extra virgin olive oil

6 cloves of garlic, minced

Procedure

1. Place the oil and garlic in a double broiler.

2. Warm over a low flame for about 2 hours.

3. Turn off the heat.

4. Cover the broiler and let sit for at least an hour (maximum overnight).

5. Strain and allow it to cool down to warm.

6. Store it in a dropper bottle.

7. Put 2 - 3 drops in the affected ear.

This oil stays good for 2 months. Just make sure to keep it in the refrigerator when not in use.

Herbal Treatment for Flu

This is simple and easy recipe to treat flu. This ale is also effective in the treatment of cold, cough, congestion and sore throat.

Things Needed

1 tsp of ground ginger

1 quart of water

2 cloves of garlic, minced

1 lemon, juiced

Pinch of cayenne pepper

Honey, to taste

Procedure

1. Bring the quart of water to boil over a medium-low flame.

2. When the water is fully boiled, reduce the flame to a low simmer.

3. Add garlic, cayenne and ginger to the hot water.

4. Cover and let sit for 20 minutes.

5. Pass the tea through a strainer.

6. Add honey and lemon just before drinking it.

Drink it one cup at a time. Keep the remaining tea in the refrigerator to be used later on. If you are taking it to treat fever, wrap yourself up in a blanket while or immediately after drinking it. This will stimulate the cayenne to cause sweating, and hence break fever.

Ginger Ale

This makes a homemade ginger ale that is amazingly great for digestion.

Things Needed

4 cups of water

Half cup ginger root (peeled and chopped)

1 ½ cup of sugar

Ice, as desired

Sparkling water, as required

Procedure

1. Combine water, ginger and sugar in a saucepan.

2. Cook over a medium flame while stirring constantly till the sugar is dissolved.

3. Bring it to a low boil and then allow it to summer till it is reduced to half. This should take about an hour or less.

4. Remove the pan off the flame.

5. Pass the ale through a strainer. Reserve the residues. You will need them to make *Ginger Chomps* (next recipe).

6. Allow it to cool down to room temperature, then put it in the refrigerator to chill.

7. When you are ready to use it, take it out of the refrigerator.

8. Fill ¼ of a glass with this ginger syrup, then fill it up with ice and sparkling water.

Enjoy!

Ginger Chomps

If you don't like the ginger ale, you can nibble on ginger chomps for digestion.

Things Needed

Half cup of ginger root (peeled and chopped), or the residual ginger from the previous recipe

Sugar, as required

Few drops of Ginger Ale (refer to the previous recipe)

Procedure

1. Take the residual ginger that you saved after straining the ale in the previous recipe.

2. Drizzle the ginger with a bit of white sugar. Toss to coat.

3. Add a few drops of ginger ale and stir to mix.

4. Make small tablet-sized bites of the ginger mixture and place them on a cookie sheet, slightly apart from one another.

5. Bake at 200 degrees or you can also put them in a food dehydrator, till the ginger is no longer sticky. This should take between 30 - 60 minutes, depending upon the size of your chomps.

6. Allow it to cool down for a while then store them all in an air tight container.

7. Keep it stored in the refrigerator.

The Digestion Condiment

This makes a condiment that you can take with meals to aid the digestion process. Sniffing it from a distance may also clear away your sinuses.

Things Needed

2 Tbsp of fresh lemon juice

1 (8 inch) piece of horseradish root

Procedure

1. Peel and finely grate the horseradish root.

2. Put it in an airtight jar.

3. Add lemon juice to the jar.

4. Place the lid and shake the jar vigorously to mix the lemon juice.

Store it in refrigerator.

Lavender Ale

This recipe makes lavender tea that helps relieve headache. It also strengthens the nervous system and is particularly good for people having insomnia.

Things Needed

4 tsp of lavender flowers

1 quart of water

1 - 2 tsp of Chamomile flowers

1 tsp of fresh rose petals

Procedure

1. Bring the quart of water to a boil over a medium-low flame.

2. When the water is fully boiled, turn off the flame.

3. Add lavender, rose petals and chamomile to the hot water.

4. Cover and let sit for 20 minutes.

5. Pass the tea through a strainer.

Enjoy!

Herbs de Provence

This makes a multi-purpose herb combination that you can use to make the following things:

1. Herbal tea that is a great remedy for cold and flu

2. Cough syrup

3. Herbal steam to clear away chest congestion

Things Needed

2 Tbsp of dried marjoram (substitute: 1 Tbsp of oregano)

5 Tbsp of dried thyme

1 ½ Tbsp of dried lavender flowers

3 Tbsp of dried savory

5 Tbsp of dried rosemary

Procedure

1. Combine all these herbs.

2. Store in an airtight container in a cool and dark place.

Herbal Steam Therapy

This steam therapy helps open up bronchioles and clears away phlegm.

Things Needed

2 quarts of water

4 tsp of Herbs de Provence (refer to previous recipe)

Procedure

1. Bring water to boil over a medium-low flame.

2. When the water is fully boiled, reduce it to a low simmer.

3. When the water is at a low simmer, turn off the flame.

4. Add Herbs de Provence to the simmering hot water. Stir to mix.

5. Cover and let sit for 10 minutes.

6. Take steam from this water by placing a towel over your head and bringing your face directly over the herbal water. Be careful with the hot pot and maintain a safe distance from the water.

7. Inhale and exhale gently for a few minutes.

8. Do not expose yourself to cool or open air immediately after taking steam.

Herbal Oral Electrolyte Solution

This recipe makes a tasty homemade oral electrolyte solution that you can drink when you are feeling physically drained of energy, low sugar level or low blood pressure.

Things Needed

> 1 tsp of baking soda
>
> 1(¼ oz.) packet of lemonade mix or Kool-Aid (unsweetened)
>
> 2 quarts of water
>
> Half tsp of salt
>
> 7 tsp of sugar
>
> Ice cubes

Procedure

1. Combine all the ingredients.

2. Drink chilled.

It stays good in the refrigerator up to 3 days, do not store it more than this.

Tea to Relieve Nausea

This tea helps relieve gastritis, nausea and indigestion.

Things Needed

1 tsp of ground nutmeg

1 ½ cups of water

Honey, to taste (optional)

Few drops of fresh lemon juice

Procedure

1. Bring water to low simmer over a medium-low flame.

2. Add the ground nutmeg to the simmering water. Cover and let sit for 15 - 20 minutes.

3. Pass the tea through a strainer.

4. Add honey and lemon just before drinking it.

Caution: Do not consume more than 5 Tablespoons of nutmeg in a day. It can become toxic and may cause severe health issues.

Headache Ale

This tea soothes the nervous system and is great to ease migraines, headaches and tiredness.

Things Needed

> 1 tsp of peppermint leaf (substitute: 1 peppermint leaf tea bag)
>
> 1 tsp of chamomile flowers (substitute: 1 chamomile tea bag)
>
> 1 quart water
>
> 1 tsp of lavender flowers (substitute: 1 lavender tea bag)
>
> 1 tsp of rosemary

Procedure

1. Bring the quart of water to boil over a medium-low flame.

2. When the water is fully boiled, turn off the flame.

3. Add chamomile. Lavender, rosemary and peppermint to the hot water. Cover and let sit for 15 - 20 minutes.

4. Pass the tea through a strainer.

5. Drink a warm cup of this tea after every 4 hours.

Herbal Balms and Ointments

Cayenne Oil

This recipe makes an anti-rheumatic, anti-inflammatory and anti-spasmodic oil that you can apply over sore muscles, sports wounds and arthritic injuries.

Things Needed

¼ cup of cayenne pepper

1 tsp of dried ginger

1 cup of extra virgin olive oil

1 tsp of ground turmeric

Procedure

1. Combine the cayenne and olive oil in a double broiler.

2. Bring it to a simmer at medium heat.

3. Let it simmer at a low flame for 2 - 3 hours.

4. Strain and rub the oil over the affected part.

Herbal Anti Fungal Treatment

This dry powdered remedy is great at treating skin rashes and fungal infections. In case of severe rashes, it may even take up to two weeks to heal.

Things Needed

1 cup cornstarch

6 tsp of boric acid

Procedure

1. Combine the cornstarch and boric acid in a large salt shaker.

2. Shake and sprinkle generously over the affected area.

Salve to Treat Pneumonia

Rubbing this salve on the back and chest works wonders in the treatment of cold and pneumonia.

Things Needed

2 oz. camphor

3 oz. powdered rosin

12 oz. lard (unsalted)

3 oz. beeswax

2 tsp of raw linseed oil

20 ml. turpentine

Procedure

1. Combine the first four ingredients in a double boiler.

2. When all the ingredients are heated through, remove the boiler off the flame.

3. Stir in the linseed oil and turpentine.

Keep stored in an airtight bottle. It stays good for years.

Herbal Mosquito Repellent

As the name suggests, this recipe makes a homemade and freshly scented mosquito repellent. Unlike the chemical-stuffed repellents, this one is not harmful for your skin.

Things Needed

15 drops of peppermint oil

1 cup of spring water

10 drops of lavender oil

Half cup of fresh lemon juice

1 shot of Vodka

Procedure

1. Combine all the ingredients in a clean sterilized spray bottle.

2. Keep it stored in the refrigerator.

3. Shake well before using.

All-In-One Ointment

This makes a multi-purpose ointment that you can apply to wounds and rashes caused by the following reasons:

1. Diaper rash
2. Insect bites
3. Pain on the wounded area
4. All kinds of itches
5. Minor wounds
6. Bleeding wounds

Things Needed

> A handful of Plantago leaves
>
> Grated beeswax, as required
>
> Olive oil, as required

Procedure

1. Coarsely chop the Plantago leaves and fill them loosely in a clean sterilized air tight jar.

2. Fill the jar up till the top with olive oil.

3. Place the cap and let sit for six weeks. Make sure the jar the away from direct sunlight.

4. After six weeks, strain and squeeze out the oil in a saucepan. Discard the herbs.

5. Add grated beeswax. You need to put one tablespoon of grated wax for each ounce of oil in the pan.

6. Heat it over a medium flame till the beeswax and oil melts, while stirring continuously.

7. Transfer it to wide-mouthed jars.

8. Allow it to cool down.

The *All-In-One Ointment* is ready to use.

Tendinitis Tincture

Apply this tincture to a soft cloth and then rub it gently over the affected area. This tincture is not suitable for pregnant women.

Things Needed

Vodka, as required

Water, as required

6 oz. dried bay leaves

Procedure

1. Put all the dried bay leaves in a 1-quart wide-mouthed jar.

2. Fill half of the jar with vodka and the remaining half with water.

3. Stir to mix.

4. Cover the jar and let sit in a cool dark place for at least 15 days (maximum 1 month). Do not forget to shake the jar once or twice every day.

5. Strain and store the tincture in a dark air tight bottle.

6. Keep it away from direct sunlight.

Homemade Pain Tincture

You can use a dropper full of this tincture after every 30 minutes, in case of chronic pain. Do not take more than 4 full droppers in a day.

Things Needed

1 tsp of St. John's Wort tincture

1 tsp of skullcap leaves tincture

Half a dropper full of ginger rhizome tincture

1 tsp of fresh oats tincture

1 tsp of Licorice root tincture

Half a dropper full of Vervain tincture

Procedure

1. Combine all the ingredients.

2. Store in a clean sterilized dropper bottle.

Marjoram Tonic

This makes an herbal homemade tonic that is great for digestion. It is also very effective and strong against the intestinal infections and bacteria.

Things Needed

1 clove of garlic, minced

2 tsp fresh marjoram (substitute: 1 tsp dried marjoram)

½ quart water

Dash of cayenne pepper

Procedure

1. Bring water to boil over a medium-low flame.

2. When the water is fully boiled, turn off the flame.

3. Add garlic, marjoram and cayenne to the hot water. Cover and let sit for 15 minutes.

4. Pass the tea through a strainer.

5. Drink half a cup after every 4 to 5 hours.

Caution: Pregnant women should not take marjoram therapeutically. Instead, you can use oregano or thyme.

Herbal Diaper Rash Ointment

This makes a soft and smooth ointment to save your baby's sensitive skin from diaper rash.

Things Needed

1 cup milk of magnesia

1 cup of corn starch

Procedure

1. Mix well both the ingredients.

2. Rub it gently and generously over the affected area.

Soothing Herbal Balm

This makes an herbal homemade soothing balm. Do not apply this over open cuts and near body orifices.

Things Needed

30 drops of clary sage essential oil

1 oz of cayenne infused oil

20 drops of cinnamon leaf essential oil

¾ oz. of beeswax

20 drops of rosemary essential oil

3 oz of goldenrod (substitute: arnica infused oil)

10 drops of sweet birch essential oil

20 drops of white camphor essential oil

Procedure

1. Melt the beeswax.

2. Stir in cayenne infused oil.

3. Allow it to cool for a while.

4. Stir in all the remaining oils. Mix well.

5. Keep it stored in a clean sterilized air tight container.

Arthritic Rub

This makes a great ointment to ease the arthritic joint pain.

Things Needed

1 tsp of dried ginger (powdered)

1 tsp of ground turmeric

Pinch of cayenne pepper

1 tsp of extra virgin olive oil, or more if the paste is too thick

Procedure

1. Combine all the ingredients to make this amazing Arthritic Rub.

2. Rub a little bit of olive area over the affected area before applying this rub, then immediately cover the skin with a few damp paper towels.

3. Do not forget to check for skin sensitivity the first you use it. Apply on a small area of skin and let stay for few hours.

Skin Soothing Gel

This makes a soothing gel that can be applied to ease the pain and inflammation caused by rashes, sunburn, razor burn, eczema, bug bites, minor wounds and scratches.

Things Needed

1 cup of fresh Aloe Vera gel

1 cup of clean fresh rose petals

Procedure

1. Combine both the ingredients in a food processor.

2. Blend well.

3. Rub it through a sieve to get the extract of rose.

This gel stays good in the refrigerator for up to 7 days.

All-Purpose Herbal Antiseptic

This makes an effective antiseptic and astringent that can be used to control acne. You can also use it as a facial toner. It can also be applied on inflammation caused by poison oak and diaper rashes.

Things Needed

A handful of clean fresh rose petals

Witch hazel extract, as required

Procedure

1. Fill a jar with rose petals. Do not cramp the petals in the jar, pack them loosely.

2. Fill the same jar with witch hazel extract. Pour in till all the roses are completely soaked in it.

3. Cover the jar with a non-metallic lid and place it in a cool and dark place. Let sit for 7 days. Make sure the jar stays away from direct sunlight and heat during this entire time.

4. Strain and transfer the liquid into a glass jar.

It stays good for months.

Recipes to Make Herbal Syrups and Tonics

Easy-To-Make Cough Syrup

This makes a sweet homemade cough syrup that can be taken by adults and kids over 2 years of age.

Things Needed

> 1 cup of honey
>
> 1 cup of fresh lemon juice
>
> 1 cup of castor oil

Procedure

1. Combine all the things. Mix well.

2. Transfer to a glass bottle or jar with a tight fitting lid.

Dosage for Adults: 1 Tablespoon during 24 hours

Dosage for Children (2 years and above): 1 teaspoon during 24 hours

The Delicious Berry Treatment

This makes a delicious berrylicious syrup to treat flu and ward off sickness.

Things Needed

Half cup of Elderberries

Half cup of honey

8 cups water

Procedure

1. Bring the water to boil.

2. Add berries to the boiling water.

3. Reduce the flame to simmer and then let it simmer till the water is reduced to two cups. This should take about 45 minutes.

4. Pass it through a strainer. Discard the berries.

5. Stir in the honey.

6. Transfer the syrup to a tight lid-container and store it in a refrigerator.

You can take this syrup a tablespoon at a time, to treat flu and sickness.

Sore Throat Syrup

This makes a cough syrup that is great for sore throats and congestion in the lungs.

Things Needed

1 tsp of thyme or sage

1 Tbsp of fresh lemon juice

6 cloves of garlic, minced

1 cup of honey

Procedure

1. Combine the thyme, garlic and honey in a double broiler, over a low flame.

2. Cook and stir till all the ingredients are thoroughly incorporated. This should take about 4 hours. Make sure you do not boil this syrup. Keep the flame to the lowest possible that is required to keep this syrup warm.

3. Pass it through a sieve. Discard the residue.

4. Stir in the lemon juice.

5. Transfer the syrup to a glass bottle or jar with a tight fitting lid

This syrup stays good for about two weeks in the refrigerator.

You can take one Tablespoon of this syrup after every 2 hours, till the symptoms ease; then four times a day.

Onion Cough Syrup

This makes an anti-bacterial cough and cold syrup. It is also very effective in the treatment sinus congestion and bronchial coughs.

Things Needed

1 large sized onion, chopped

2 tsp of minced garlic

½ tsp of ginger

Honey, as required

1 tsp of oregano

Procedure

1. Combine the onion, ginger, oregano and garlic in a double broiler, over low flame.

2. Pour in honey; it should be enough to cover both the things in the broiler.

3. Cook over low flame till the onions are translucent.

4. Let it cool for a while.

5. Strain and store the liquid in a tight-fitting lid container.

You can take one teaspoon of this syrup after every hour, till the symptoms eases; then 4 - 6 times a day.

Thyme Cough Syrup

This makes another effective honey flavored cough syrup.

Things Needed

> 3 tsp thyme leaves or lemon thyme
>
> ¼ cup of honey
>
> 1 cup of water
>
> ½ lemon, juiced

Procedure

1. Bring water to boil over medium-low flame.

2. When the water is fully boiled, turn off the flame.

3. Add thyme to the hot water. Cover and let sit for 15 - 20 minutes.

4. Pass the tea through a strainer.

5. Stir in honey and lemon juice.

Dosage for Adults: 1 Tablespoon after every hour, when symptoms are worst; then 4 - 6 times a day.

Dosage for Children: 1 teaspoon after every hour, when symptoms are worst; then 4 times a day.

Chinese Immunity Tonic

As the name suggests, this tonic is great at strengthening the immune system. While you can take it as it is, adding a bit of it in your meal, stew or soup will make it easy for you to have your entire family consume this healthy tonic.

Things Needed

1/3 oz. Dioscorea opposita yam

1/3 oz. Astragalus membranaceus root

1/3 oz. Codonopsis pilosula root

1/3 oz. lotus seed (Nelumbo nucifera)

Half cup of chopped carrots

Half cup of chopped kale

6 cups of water

Miso, to taste

Procedure

1. Combine all the herbs and water in a saucepan.

2. Boil on a medium-low flame, till the liquid is reduced by half.

3. Discard the Astragalus and Codonopsis.

4. Stir in the carrots and kale.

5. Cook till the carrots are soft.

6. Finally, stir in miso.

Final Words

Now that you know how easy herbal medicines are to make and how many diseases they can cure, why not switch to this healthier alternative cure! Not only is it harmless, it is economical, it is side effect-free, it is easy to make and most importantly, it saves your body from being antibiotic resistant.

As you may have discovered by now, the ingredients used in these recipes are all homemade things that are used on a daily basis and are almost always available in a standard kitchen pantry. So why rush to the doctor every time you cough or fall off a step? Open this book, find the right recipe and save yourself a doctor's visit.

Stay Herbal! Stay Healthy!